Staying Connected

Together We Can: Pandemic

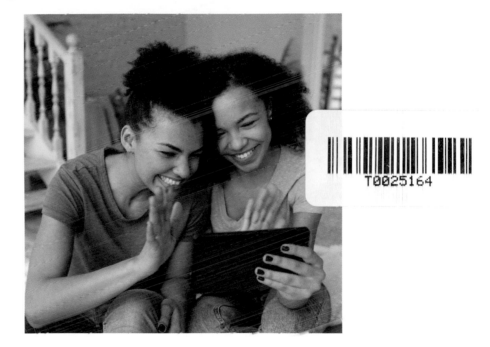

By Shannon Stocker

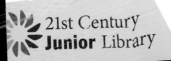

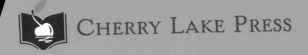

Published in the United States of America by Cherry Lake Publishing Group
Ann Arbor, Michigan
www.cherrylakepublishing.com

Reading Adviser: Marla Conn, MS, Ed., Literacy specialist, Read-Ability, Inc.

Photo Credits: © silverkblackstock/Shutterstock.com, cover, 1; © kriangkrainetnangrong/Shutterstock.com, 4; © Odua Images/Shutterstock.com, 6; © Prostock-studio/Shutterstock.com, 8; © fizkes/Shutterstock.com, 10; © Rawpixel.com/Shutterstock.com, 12; © goodluz/Shutterstock.com, 14; © CMYK/Shutterstock.com, 16; © maratr/Shutterstock.com, 18; © Aleksandr Khmeliov/Shutterstock.com, 20

Cherry Lake Press is an imprint of Cherry Lake Publishing Group.

Library of Congress Cataloging-in-Publication Data

Names: Stocker, Shannon, author.
Title: Staying connected / Shannon Stocker.
Description: Ann Arbor, Michigan : Cherry Lake Publishing, [2021] | Series: Together we can: pandemic | Includes index. | Audience: Grades 2-3 | Summary: "The COVID-19 pandemic introduced many changes into children's lives. Staying Connected gives actionable suggestions to help young readers stay in touch with friends and loved ones as we navigate the current outbreak. This book includes science content, based on current CDC recommendations, as well as social emotional content to help with personal wellness and development of empathy. All books in the 21st Century Junior Library encourage readers to think critically and creatively, and use their problem-solving skills. Book includes table of contents, sidebars, glossary, index, and author biography"—Provided by publisher.
Identifiers: LCCN 2020040010 (print) | LCCN 2020040011 (ebook) | ISBN 9781534180093 (hardcover) | ISBN 9781534181809 (paperback) | ISBN 9781534181106 (pdf) | ISBN 9781534182813 (ebook)
Subjects: LCSH: COVID-19 (Disease)—Social aspects—Juvenile literature. | Epidemics—Social aspects—Juvenile literature. | Quarantine—Social aspects—Juvenile literature. | Social interaction—Juvenile literature.
Classification: LCC RA644.C67 S764 2021 (print) | LCC RA644.C67 (ebook) | DDC 614.5/92414—dc23
LC record available at https://lccn.loc.gov/2020040010
LC ebook record available at https://lccn.loc.gov/2020040011

Cherry Lake Publishing Group would like to acknowledge the work of the Partnership for 21st Century Learning, a Network of Battelle for Kids. Please visit http://www.battelleforkids.org/networks/p21 for more information.

Printed in the United States of America
Corporate Graphics

CONTENTS

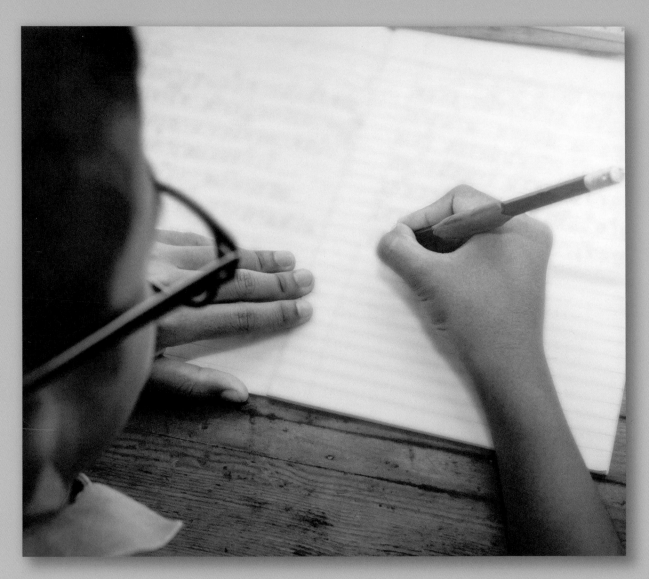

Stay connected with your feelings by keeping a journal.

Staying Connected with You!

When the **coronavirus pandemic** swept the world, everyone felt many of the same emotions. The possibility of getting sick created fear and anxiety. Being **quarantined** at home left people feeling confused, sad, and lonely. All of these feelings can be overwhelming when you feel trapped inside. Staying connected with your friends and family can help decrease these emotions. But how do you stay connected when you also have to stay apart?

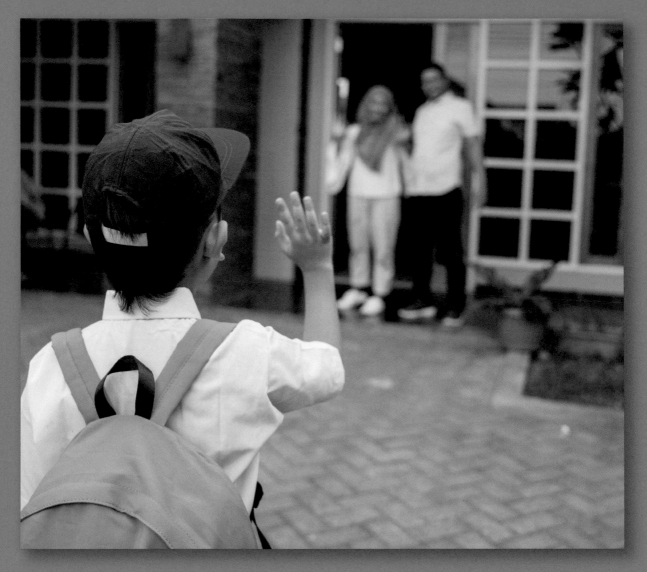

Greeting neighbors from a safe distance makes everyone happy!

Staying connected with your own emotions in a healthy way is also important. Doctors agree that this helps our brains work better. Take time every day to **validate** your feelings by asking yourself open-ended questions. *How am I feeling today? How big are my feelings? What am I feeling right now? What can I do to make today better?*

Ask Questions!

How do you think adults around you feel about pandemics? Ask them!

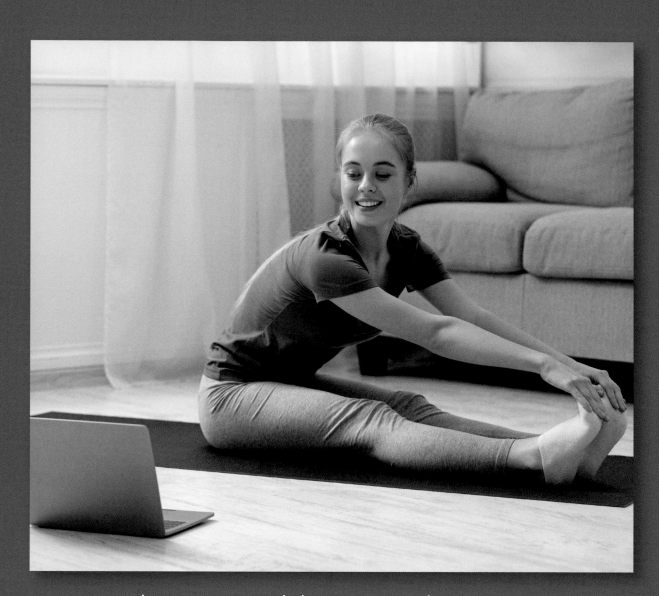

Online yoga sessions help us connect with our emotions.
The exercise is great for our bodies too!

When the coronavirus first hit, everyone's life changed. Maybe you suddenly stopped going to school. Maybe you are homeschooled but could no longer play with friends. New routines are important during times like this. **Predictability** helps us feel safe and secure. Establishing goals can also help you feel more confident and independent.

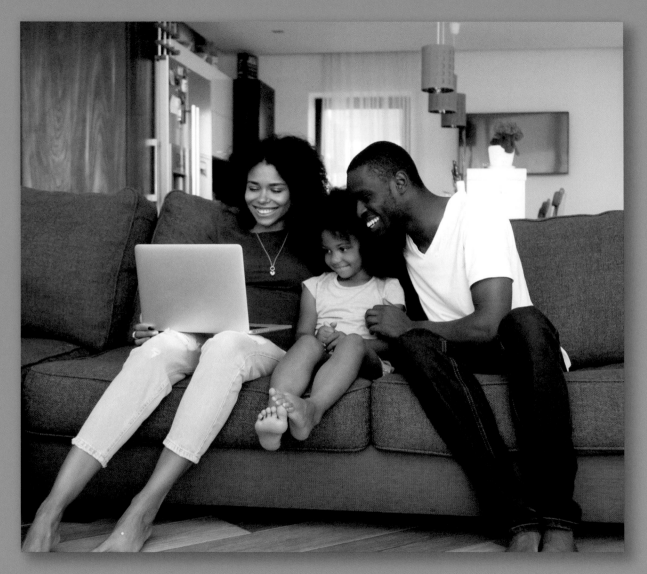

Use technology like Skype, phones, FaceTime, or Zoom
to visit with friends and family members.

Staying Connected with Friends and Family

Have you ever heard of **empathy**? If you've ever felt sad when a friend was hurt, that's empathy. We bond with other people when we share emotions. It might be harder to stay connected with friends and family when we can't be with them. But we can still feel empathy for them, even when we're far apart. We can use this opportunity to connect with the people we love.

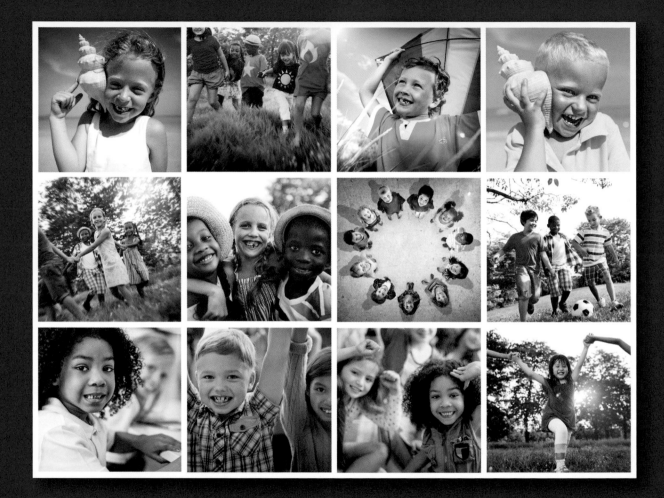

Look through old photos and talk about your favorite memories.

Have you ever received a letter in the mail? It feels great! Writing letters can be a powerful way to connect with a friend, family member, or teacher. It gives that person a **tangible** thing to look at and hold, and it will always remind them of you. You can write letters or draw pictures to say thank you, happy birthday, or that you're thinking of them.

Think!

What kinds of things could you make that would fit in an envelope to be sent through the mail?

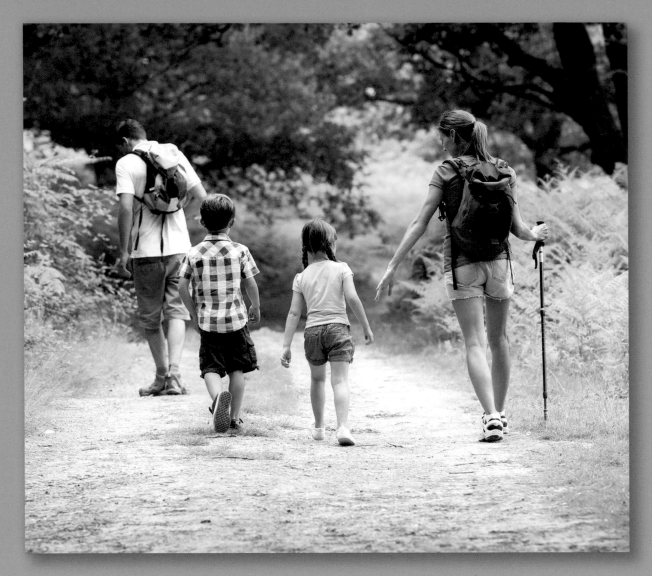

Hiking with family is a great way to connect with nature.

Staying Connected with the World

Although big groups can't gather during a pandemic, it is safe to go outside. Did you know our bodies get healthy doses of vitamin D from the sun? Being in nature can also bring a sense of calm and reduce anxiety. Take time to appreciate the birds, flowers, and trees around you. There are lots of phone apps that can help you identify different types of plants too.

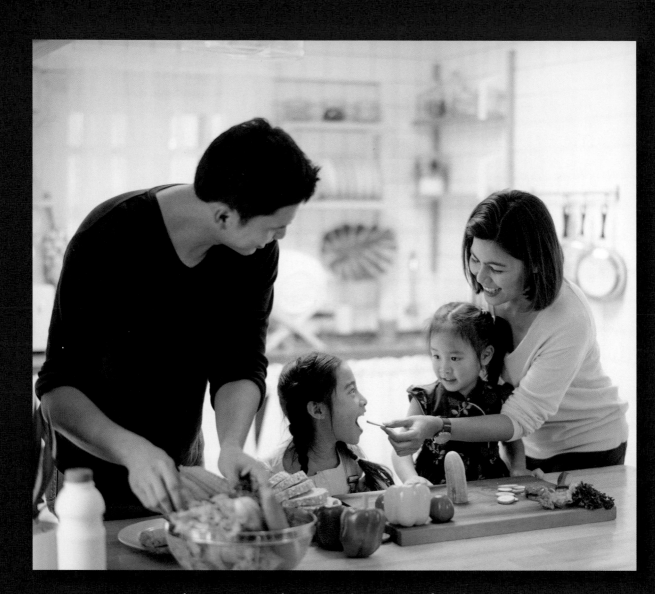

Learning to cook a new meal is something your family can do together.

Just because you're stuck inside doesn't mean you can't learn something new about the world! Spin a globe, close your eyes, and let your finger land. Learn a fun fact about that country. Or find a yummy recipe **indigenous** to that region and ask an adult to help you make it. Remember that people in that country are facing the pandemic too.

Look!

How many different kinds of plants can you find near your home?

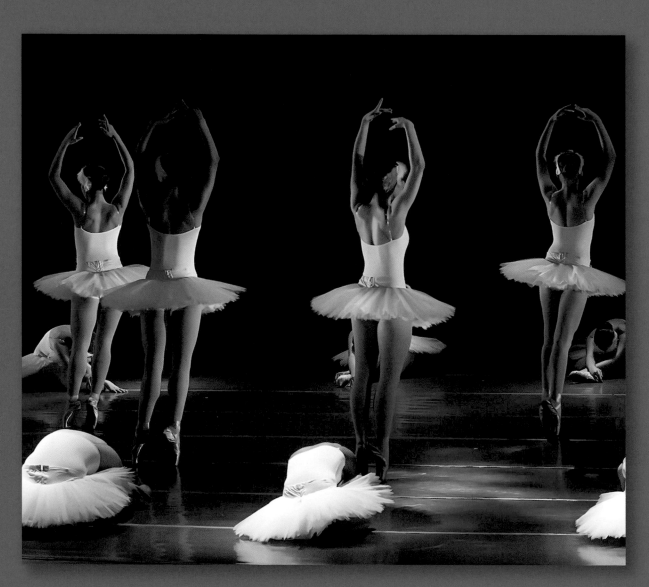

Watch a ballet performance online!

With travel around the world limited, many places have made **virtual** field trips available online for free. Use your time at home to connect with things you love. Are you an animal fan? Visit a zoo that's thousands of miles away! Do you like art? Go to a museum in France! From Disney World rides to digital libraries, the options are (virtually!) endless.

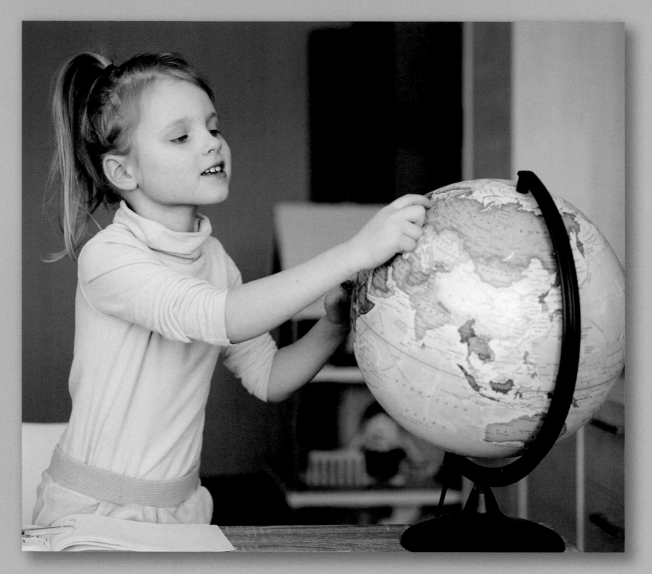

What part of the world is your family from? Learn more about it online!

Think about the big, wide world in which we live. There is so much to see and learn. There are so many types of cultures, places, and people. During a pandemic, we have the time to slow down. We can reflect on our feelings, reach out to those we love, and learn something new. We have so many options to stay connected.

What will you choose today?

GLOSSARY

coronavirus (kuh-ROH-nuh-vye-ruhs) a family of viruses that cause a variety of illnesses in people and other mammals

empathy (EM-puh-thee) the ability to understand and share another person's feelings

indigenous (in-DIH-juh-nuhs) originating from, or characteristic of, a particular region

pandemic (pan-DEM-ik) an outbreak of a disease that affects a large part of the population

predictability (prih-dikt-uh-BIL-uh-tee) the ability to know what to expect because of repeated actions or behaviors

quarantined (KWOR-uhn-teend) isolated from others

tangible (TAN-jih-buhl) something that can be touched

validate (VAL-ih-dayt) to support or recognize something as worthy, true, or valuable

virtual (VUR-choo-uhl) accessed by a computer, especially online

FIND OUT MORE

WEBSITES

AwesomeJelly—The 8 Best Apps to Identify Unknown Plants and Flowers
https://awesomejelly.com/8-best-apps-identify-unknown-plants-flowers-2

Google Arts & Culture—Collections
https://artsandculture.google.com/partner?hl=en

Mommy Poppins—Best Games Kids Can Play on Zoom Virtually with Friends
https://mommypoppins.com/boredom-busters/fun-games-kids-play-with-friends-virtually

NEAToday—Social-Emotional Learning Should Be Priority During COVID-19 Crisis
http://neatoday.org/2020/04/15/social-emotional-learning-during-covid

Today—Virtual Field Trips You Can Take from Home
https://www.today.com/parents/try-these-virtual-field-trips-educational-fun-home-t176105

INDEX

ABOUT THE AUTHOR

Shannon Stocker writes picture books, books for young readers, and *Chicken Soup* stories. She loves staying connected by taking daily nature walks, doing yoga, playing online guessing games with friends, and helping her children stay in touch with new pen pals. Shannon lives in Louisville, Kentucky, with Greg, Cassidy, Tye, and far too many critters.